COVID-19 and the Challenges
OF THE NEW NORMAL

Marcia S. Gresko

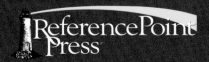
ReferencePoint
Press

San Diego, CA

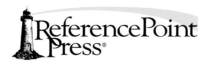
ReferencePoint
Press®

About the Author

Marcia S. Gresko has written more than a dozen books for children and young adults on a variety of social studies and science topics. For eighteen years she worked for an educational toy company developing products from board games to electronic learning aids. She has also taught students in grade levels from preschool to high school. She lives in Southern California.

© 2021 ReferencePoint Press, Inc.
Printed in the United States

For more information, contact:
ReferencePoint Press, Inc.
PO Box 27779
San Diego, CA 92198
www.ReferencePointPress.com

ALL RIGHTS RESERVED.
No part of this work covered by the copyright hereon may be reproduced or used in any form or by any means—graphic, electronic, or mechanical, including photocopying, recording, taping, web distribution, or information storage retrieval systems—without the written permission of the publisher.

Picture Credits:
Cover: Pixfly/iStock

8: primipil/iStock
12: Larry Marano/Newscom
15: Matt Gush/Shutterstock.com
19: Associated Press
23: martinedoucet/iStock

27: sirtravelalot/Shutterstock
30: Associated Press
35: Andrea Migliarini/iStock
37: blackCAT/iStock
43: Maury Aaseng
48: zstock/Shutterstock
53: FatCamera/iStock

LIBRARY OF CONGRESS CATALOGING-IN-PUBLICATION DATA

Names: Gresko, Marcia S., author.
Title: COVID-19 and the challenges of the new normal / by Marcia S. Gresko.
Description: San Diego, CA : ReferencePoint Press, Inc., 2021. | Series: Understanding the COVID-19 pandemic | Includes bibliographical references and index.
Identifiers: LCCN 2020046307 (print) | LCCN 2020046308 (ebook) | ISBN 9781678200329 (library binding) | ISBN 9781678200336 (ebook)
Subjects: LCSH: COVID-19 Pandemic, 2020--Juvenile literature. | Social change--History--21st century--Juvenile literature. | Social history--21st century--Juvenile literature.
Classification: LCC HM831 .G74 2021 (print) | LCC HM831 (ebook) | DDC 362.1962/414--dc23
LC record available at https://lccn.loc.gov/2020046307
LC ebook record available at https://lccn.loc.gov/2020046308

CONTENTS

The COVID-19 Pandemic:
The First Nine Months of 2020

January

(11) China reports first known death from mysterious virus that infected dozens in Wuhan in December.

(20) WHO reports that Japan, South Korea, and Thailand have first confirmed virus cases outside of mainland China.

(30) WHO declares global health emergency.

(31) US restricts travel from China.

February

(2) Philippines reports first coronavirus death outside of China.

(5) Japan quarantines *Diamond Princess* cruise ship; within 2 weeks the ship has more than 600 infections.

(11) WHO names the disease caused by the new coronavirus COVID-19 (for *co*rona*v*irus *d*isease 20*19*).

(23) Europe's first major outbreak occurs in Italy.

(26) Brazil has Latin America's first known case of coronavirus.

March

(13) US president Donald Trump officially declares national emergency.

(19) California becomes first US state to enact statewide shutdown.

(24) Officials announce 1-year postponement of 2020 Tokyo Summer Olympics.

(26) US becomes world leader in confirmed coronavirus infections.

(27) President Trump signs $2 trillion economic stimulus bill sent to him by Congress.

April

(2) Pandemic shutdowns have cost nearly 10 million Americans their jobs.

(10) Coronavirus cases surge in Russia.

(14) IMF warns of worst global downturn since Great Depression.

(17) President Trump encourages protests of social distancing restrictions.

(26) Pandemic has killed more than 200,000 and sickened more than 2.8 million worldwide.

(30) Several major airlines begin requiring face masks.

May

(1) FDA authorizes remdesivir as an emergency treatment for COVID-19.

(17) Japan and Germany fall into recession.

(26) Widespread protests begin after George Floyd is killed by Minneapolis police; because many protesters wear masks, feared virus outbreaks do not occur.

(27) US has more than 100,000 COVID-19 deaths, surpassing all other nations.

June

(4) Previously spared regions of Middle East, Latin America, Africa, and South Asia have large spikes.

(11) Coronavirus cases in Africa exceed 200,000, with one-fourth in South Africa.

(20) Florida and South Carolina are among 19 US states experiencing sharp rise in new infections.

(28) Final phase of clinical trials for AstraZeneca–University of Oxford COVID-19 vaccine begins in Brazil.

July

(11) For the first time, President Trump wears a mask during a public appearance.

(16) Georgia's governor rescinds local government mask mandates.

(17) After easing restrictions in May, skyrocketing infections force India to reimpose lockdown.

(27) Final phase of clinical trials for Moderna COVID-19 vaccine begins in the US.

August

(9) New Zealand achieves 100 days without a new diagnosis of coronavirus.

(11) Amid global skepticism, Russia announces first approved-for-use coronavirus vaccine.

(17) Democrats begin first-ever, all-virtual convention to nominate the party's presidential candidate, Joe Biden.

(23) FDA authorizes convalescent plasma as an emergency treatment for COVID-19.

(27) Before a crowd of about 1,500 people, President Trump accepts Republican presidential nomination.

September

(8) Nine of the leading drug companies developing COVID-19 vaccines pledge in writing to put safety before speed.

(21) President Trump tells supporters at an Ohio rally that COVID "affects virtually nobody."

(30) The pandemic has killed more than 1 million people and sickened nearly 34 million worldwide. In the US, the pandemic has killed nearly 207,000 people and sickened more than 7 million. Two days later, on October 2, President Trump tweets that he and First Lady Melania Trump have tested positive for the virus that causes COVID-19.

Based on Derrick Bryson Taylor, "A Timeline of the Coronavirus Pandemic," *New York Times*, July 21, 2020. www.nytimes.com.

The Crisis Begins

The Huanan Seafood Wholesale Market stretches over 12 acres (4.9 ha) in Wuhan, a city in central China. With more than one thousand vendors, the market is a busy, crowded place. In addition to its huge selection of fish and shellfish, in the winter of 2019, one market section offered seventy-five species of wild animals. Customers could choose from beavers and bats to snakes and scaly, anteater-like pangolins, available to be freshly slaughtered. These conditions created an environment in which viruses could spread between species. It is here, researchers believe, that a new, or novel, coronavirus spread to humans and led to the disease that became known as COVID-19.

Events moved quickly. On December 31, 2019, China announced a cluster of cases of a pneumonia-like illness in Wuhan. Three weeks later, China placed the city of 11 million people under quarantine. By then the virus had already spread beyond Wuhan—and beyond China's borders.

On January 30, 2020, with more than nine thousand cases reported internationally in eighteen countries, the World Health Organization (WHO) announced a global public health emergency. Less than two months later, on March 13 the WHO declared the European continent the pandemic's epicenter, with more cases and deaths than all affected countries, besides China, combined.

Italy was among the hardest-hit countries in Europe, prompting a nearly monthlong lockdown that began on March 9. It was essentially a nationwide quarantine. More than 60 million people stayed home.

The Crisis in the United States

To stem the spread in the United States, President Donald Trump ordered a series of travel bans and restrictions. On March 13 he declared a national state of emergency, freeing up $50 billion to help fight the pandemic. The announcement came the same day Idaho announced its first confirmed case of coronavirus, making it the forty-ninth US state to report being affected. By that date, the number of US cases had topped twenty-two hundred, and forty-nine people had died.

But the crisis was just beginning. Schools and colleges across the country began to close. Several states postponed their presidential primaries. Sports leagues canceled or suspended play. Iconic events, like New York City's St. Patrick's Day Parade and the Boston Marathon, were scratched.

The Centers for Disease Control and Prevention (CDC) recommended in March against gatherings of fifty or more people. That quickly became warnings against gatherings of more than ten people. Nonessential businesses, from theaters to retail stores, closed. Recreational and cultural attractions, from parks to museums, ceased operation. Television shows and films halted production. Even houses of worship shut their doors.

By March 25 governors in all but five states had issued stay-at-home orders for their residents. By mid-April, shutdown declarations were in effect in all fifty states.

A massive wave of unemployment swept the nation. Millions of mostly blue-collar workers in shuttered industries were laid off. White-collar workers who still had jobs mostly worked from home. Essential workers serving grocery stores, driving public transportation, and caring for the sick in hospitals and nursing homes stayed the course.

The Struggle for Normalcy

For much of 2020, daily life was anything but normal. The spring months, marking the start of the pandemic, were chaotic. Panicked supermarket shoppers endured long lines and packed

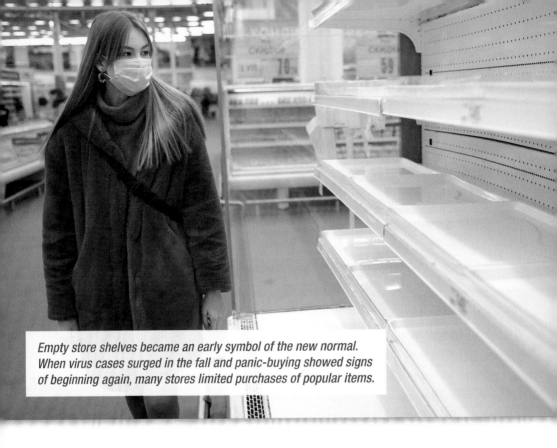

Empty store shelves became an early symbol of the new normal. When virus cases surged in the fall and panic-buying showed signs of beginning again, many stores limited purchases of popular items.

aisles to stock up on staples, stripping shelves of toilet paper and water, flour, and spaghetti. Disinfectants and cold and flu medicines were sold out. Even into fall, grocery stores were preparing special pandemic pallets—wooden structures stockpiled with high-demand products, from cleaning supplies to dried pasta—in anticipation of the next surge.

From the beginning, the medical response to the crisis was lacking. On the front lines, testing was inadequate. The personal protective equipment (PPE) needed by medical professionals and health care workers was scarce. Lifesaving ventilators for those afflicted with COVID-19 were in limited supply. Hospital parking lots became morgues. While some improvements were made by fall, a third wave of the virus in the Midwest and Great Plains states threatened to strain resources and overcome hospitals in those regions. In October, Wisconsin opened a 530-bed field hospital at the state's fairgrounds outside Milwaukee to help deal with the rising numbers of COVID cases.

Mitigation efforts seemed powerless to stop the spread, even as the president predicted, "It's going to disappear. One day—it's like a miracle—it will disappear."[1] Public health officials called on the nation to practice social distancing, keeping a minimum of 6 feet (1.8 m) from others. This would flatten the curve, or slow the infection rate, enabling health care systems to cope with the outbreak without being overwhelmed.

But the crisis deepened. Millions have suffered, but it is clear that communities of color have borne the brunt of the disease and its economic fallout. A disproportionate number of people of color have gotten sick and died from the virus. Job losses have also been greater in these communities.

As the pandemic wore on, temporary government aid to help people and businesses weather the economic storm ran out. In an effort to open the economy, some states, even some badly hit by the virus, loosened restrictions. Businesses in many parts of the country re-opened, and schools made plans to do the same. As health experts predicted, cases spiked. That spike forced some cities and states to reinstate temporary shutdowns and restrictions, but the numbers continued to rise. A third spike began in October, and by the end of the month, according to the Johns Hopkins Coronavirus Resource Center, the United States had more than 9 million cases and nearly 230,000 deaths—the highest numbers of any nation on earth.

> "It's going to disappear. One day—it's like a miracle—it will disappear."[1]
>
> —Donald Trump, forty-fifth president of the United States

Since the virus emerged in Wuhan, it has spread to more than two hundred countries and territories. As of October, it appeared that coronavirus and its new normal would be around for a while. Although the situation has been discouraging, many experts in fields from health care to education to social justice believe the new normal presents an opportunity for a different and perhaps better normal.

CHAPTER ONE

The Workplace

Throughout much of 2020, desperate Americans lined up for miles outside drive-through food pantries. Rents went unpaid. Household savings, if there were any, were strained.

Because of the nationwide shutdown, the US economy collapsed. The Bureau of Labor Statistics estimated that 20.5 million Americans lost their jobs in April. The unemployment rate soared to 14.7 percent, the highest level since the Great Depression. Hardest hit were restaurants, hotels, and retail stores. Manufacturing workers, white-collar and government personnel, and even health care workers were also laid off.

During the summer and early fall, employment numbers bounced back more quickly than some experts predicted as businesses began phased reopening. The Bureau of Labor Statistics jobs report for September showed that unemployment fell to 7.9 percent. However, the report noted that progress had slowed, and there were signs that many job losses would be long term or permanent.

Hernan Gonzalez, a fifty-eight-year old hospitality worker, has worked in the hospitality industry for forty years. He was laid off in March after sixteen years as an employee of the Diplomat Hotel in Hollywood, Florida. He has not worked since. His health care benefits ran out in October. "I'm hoping next year I can get my job back," he said. "But with the way things are happening, I don't see that window that's going to guarantee that I'm going to have a job next year."[2]

Disproportionate Pain

Not everyone has been equally affected by the crushing economic crisis. Communities of color, low-income households, individuals with less education, and women have borne the brunt of the losses.

Job losses have been greatest among people of color and the poor, many of whom were employed in the devastated industries. According to the US Department of Labor, April unemployment, which rose to the highest rate since the pandemic began, was 18.9 percent for Hispanics, 16.7 percent for African Americans, 14.5 percent for Asians, and 14.2 percent for Caucasians. Lower-wage workers making fifteen dollars per hour or less suffered an employment decline of 35 percent. In contrast, higher wage earners in positions where earnings topped thirty-two dollars per hour experienced job losses of just 9 percent, according to payroll processing company ADP.

Education was also a factor, according to the US Department of Labor report. The April unemployment rate for workers with a bachelor's degree or higher was 8.4 percent. Workers with some college had an unemployment rate of 15 percent. But workers with only a high school degree had a whopping 17.3 percent unemployment rate—more than double that of college graduates. For those without a high school diploma, the rate was even higher—21.2 percent.

Gender played a role as well. "I think we should go ahead and call this a 'shecession,'"[3] said C. Nicole Mason, head of a women's think tank. According to the Bureau of Labor Statistics, women accounted for 55 percent of the 20.5 million jobs lost in April. Women's unemployment was nearly three points higher than men's, the largest gap since the Great Recession. Experts noted that this was partly due to the highest employment declines being in sectors with greater female employment. But another important factor was likely child care, as schools and day care facilities closed and many women stayed home to care for their children. By September, with nearly half of school districts opening virtually, women left the workforce at four times the rate men did, the US Department of Labor reported. Youli Lee, a federal worker in Fairfax, Virginia, was one of them. Working remotely from home, with three young boys attending virtual school, was exhausting. "I can't keep this up. This is too much,"[4] she realized. She took a leave of absence.

Government Aid

Amid mounting unemployment and economic disruption, Congress stepped in, passing two economic relief packages in early March. Most importantly, at the end of the month, Congress passed the $2 trillion Coronavirus Aid, Relief, and Economic Security Act. As a result of the act, many Americans received a one-time cash payment amounting to about $1,200. In addition, the act made significant changes to unemployment assistance, increasing the benefits and who was eligible. Most unemployed workers received an additional $600 a week from the federal government. That benefit ended in July.

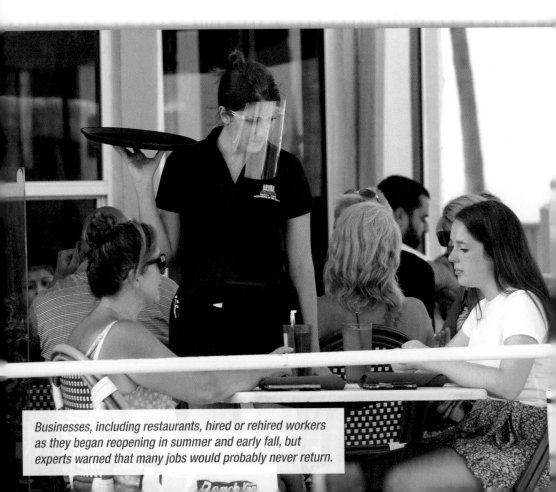

Businesses, including restaurants, hired or rehired workers as they began reopening in summer and early fall, but experts warned that many jobs would probably never return.

As money for rent and food ran out, workers scrambled to find jobs. Like millions of others, Nick Lancaster, an information technology support analyst, lost his job of seventeen years in April. Job hunting was tough. There was lots of competition, and interviews were held remotely. It took him four months and two hundred applications to find a new job. According to a New York Federal Reserve survey in July, Americans felt they had a less than 50 percent chance of finding a new job within three months if they lost their job during the crisis. They were likely correct. An Economic Policy Institute blog in July revealed that there were 14 million more unemployed workers than there were job openings, so millions were unlikely to find jobs regardless of how hard they tried. Jacob Perlman, laid off from his job as a housekeeper at a fitness club, said that if there were jobs out there, he would take one. In the meantime, like so many others, he waits to see what will happen.

Essential Workers

Throughout much of 2020, millions of workers hunkered down at home either because they had lost their jobs or because they could work from home. But millions of other workers remained on the front lines every day. These men and women were deemed essential workers.

State governors issued executive orders identifying the vital industries and essential workers in their states. In the face of the crisis, health care providers—doctors, nurses, pharmacists, orderlies, technicians, and custodians in hospitals and caregivers in nursing homes—worked grueling hours. Food production and delivery workers—including farmers, meatpackers, truckers, warehouse laborers, and grocery store clerks—pulled punishing shifts. Law enforcement and public safety professionals, such as police officers and firefighters, remained vigilant. Utility workers made sure the electricity stayed on and water streamed from faucets; sanitation workers ensured trash was collected. Mail carriers delivered mail—from critical medications to Social Security checks. Public transportation workers, such as bus drivers

Remote Work Is Here to Stay

What began as a pandemic-produced necessity—working remotely—is likely here to stay. Companies such as Ford Motor Company, Google, and Target have told employees to continue working from home at least until the summer of 2021. Other companies—including Facebook, Microsoft, Shopify, and outdoor recreation and clothing retailer REI—have all announced some form of permanent remote work option as the new normal. Even some traditional businesses, like Nationwide Mutual Insurance Company, are offering thousands of their employees the opportunity to work from home permanently.

Jack Dorsey, chief executive officer of Twitter, has been vocal in his support of having employees work from home, saying, "If you're in a role and situation that enables you to work from home and you want to continue, do so . . . forever if you want." Twitter employees seem happy to take him up on it. In a company survey, most employees felt they were more productive from their home offices, and 70 percent wanted to continue to work remotely at least three days a week.

But not all companies were following this example. Banking industry giant JPMorgan Chase called all of its remote workers back into the office at the end of September. The company cited productivity concerns and the difficulty of maintaining a corporate culture.

Quoted in Elizabeth Dwoskin, "Americans Might Never Come Back to the Office, and Twitter Is Leading the Charge," *Washington Post*, October 1, 2020. www.washingtonpost.com.

and subway operators, shuttled essential workers to and from their shifts. As one hospital worker whose brother is a manager at a pharmacy and whose father is a dispatcher for a police department said, "I guess we all just feel our work is important. People need food. They need medicine. They need to feel safe. Our approach is 'These jobs have to get done and we're going to do them.'"[5]

According to a Brookings Institution analysis, approximately 90 million people are employed in American industries that are defined as essential by the US Department of Homeland Security. While essential workers are a large and diverse group, they share some demographic characteristics. According to a study by the Economic Policy Institute, people of color account for 43 percent of all essential workers in the nation. A majority do not hold a college degree. Three-quarters work for below-average wages, and most have a household income of $40,000 or less. Author and researcher Andre Perry wonders whether such workers should be called "heroes or hostages. They deserve our credit and our admiration, but it's not like they have a choice here." He added, "Go to work or starve."[6]

"I guess we all just feel our work is important. People need food. They need medicine. They need to feel safe. Our approach is 'These jobs have to get done and we're going to do them.'"[5]

—New York City hospital worker

Dangerous Work

The people doing the jobs that have kept America functioning during the pandemic have encountered dangers that no one could have anticipated. Many essential workers have sacrificed

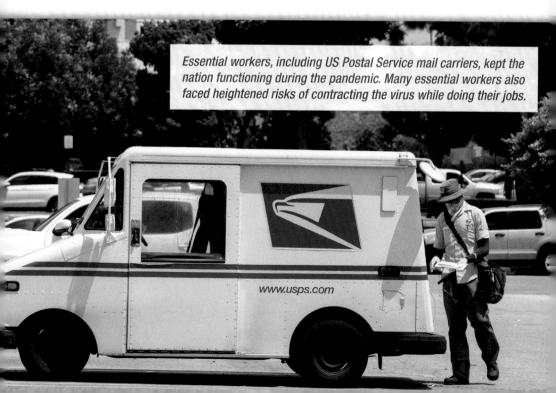

Essential workers, including US Postal Service mail carriers, kept the nation functioning during the pandemic. Many essential workers also faced heightened risks of contracting the virus while doing their jobs.

their own health and put their families at risk of contracting the virus. Some workers paid with their lives. The mortality rate of essential workers has been many times higher than that of professional and office workers.

Several factors have endangered workers. Foremost among them is repeated exposure at work. For example, according to a study by the University of Washington School of Public Health, more than 77 percent of health care workers, from doctors to home health aides, have been exposed to infectious diseases at least once a week. In addition, there have been shocking shortages of the PPE needed by these workers. In the face of the highly contagious virus, workers have scrounged for equipment,

Learning to Defuse Conflict Over Masks

Store workers, from grocery clerks to retail associates, have had to contend with more than stocking shelves and tidying dressing rooms during the pandemic. As state and local governments have mandated masks, and markets and shops have instituted "no mask, no service" rules to protect their employees and their customers, these workers have become the policy enforcers.

While most people have accepted mask wearing as the new normal, some have not—leading to tense, even violent confrontations. A Target employee in Van Nuys, California, ended up with a broken arm. A convenience store cashier in Perkasie, Pennsylvania, was punched three times in the face.

Now some retail workers have been learning a new skill—conflict management—designed to help them navigate the new normal. The online training, a collaboration between the National Retail Federation and the Crisis Prevention Institute, highlights common scenarios such as asking a customer to wear a mask and dealing with customers who are upset that fellow shoppers are flouting mask rules.

Restaurant workers have endured similar treatment, prompting their trade group to introduce training starting in September 2020. The aim is to help workers defuse conflict when dealing with angry diners who refuse to wear masks and follow other restrictions.

fund-raised for PPE, or paid for it out of their own pockets. Some have even repurposed items such as trash bags and raincoats to shield themselves.

Increased workloads and mounting stress have contributed to the dire situation. According to the interactive database Lost on the Frontline, a partnership between Kaiser Health News and the *Guardian*, as of August, more than nine hundred health care workers had died of COVID-19. Most of them were nurses.

Grocery store workers have also worked in fear, filling shelves and keeping the checkout lines going. About 3 million people work in the nation's approximately forty thousand grocery stores. While the general public have been advised to visit the grocery store as infrequently as possible, these workers have risked contagion daily. In the first weeks of the pandemic, grocery stores did not provide employees with PPE, nor did they require shoppers to wear masks, prompting workers at various chains to walk off the job or call in sick in protest. A long-time grocery store clerk in a suburb of New York said, "The first week when people were panic buying, it felt like a war zone. We were scrambling to get people in place. We didn't have gloves, masks or anything. People were on top of each other. People were complaining. People were upset there was no toilet paper or paper towels. . . . It was turmoil."[7] In the first one hundred days of the pandemic, more than 11,500 grocery workers were infected or exposed to the virus, and more than 80 died, according to the United Food and Commercial Workers International Union.

Since then, improvements to working conditions have been made at many grocery stores. Plexiglas barriers between cashiers and customers have been installed. Floor markers placed every 6 feet (1.8 m) in checkout lines have obliged customers

> "The first week when people were panic buying, it felt like a war zone. We were scrambling to get people in place. We didn't have gloves, masks or anything."[7]
>
> —Suburban New York grocery store clerk

to observe social distancing rules. And while issues have arisen, most grocery stores have been enforcing mask requirements for both employees and customers.

But even into the fall, outbreaks continued at some grocery stores. In Riverside County, California, for example, grocery stores were the source of the highest number of COVID-19 outbreaks—forty-eight—from July through September.

White-Collar Workers

While many workers in retail, service, and manufacturing jobs have not been able to perform their work remotely, or even manage to safely socially distance during their workday, most white-collar workers have been able to work from home. Bedrooms have become offices. Kitchen tables have served as desks. Meetings have been held over Zoom, an online platform for video and audio communication. Employees often appear to be dressed in work attire, but below the waist, they are wearing pajamas. Zoom meetings have also included barking dogs, flushing toilets, and toddlers teetering around unfazed.

A Brookings Institution report indicated that about half of employed adults in the United States were working from home in the early days of the pandemic. By September, according to the Bureau of Labor Statistics, that number had shrunk to about 23 percent. Some big companies, such as Google, however, planned to allow their employees to work remotely until well into 2021.

But remote work has challenges too. A survey of nearly three thousand office workers across all fifty states at the end of March revealed some of them. Survey respondents noted technical troubles, difficulty effectively communicating with others, the inability to find important information needed to do their jobs, household distractions, and juggling family responsibilities. Also mentioned was feeling disconnected from work colleagues and a sense of loneliness and isolation, leading to overall job dissatisfaction. In October, Ashley Fetters, a journalist for the *Washington Post* who has been reporting from home since the pandemic began, wrote a piece on the loneliness of remote work. Looking toward a future when the

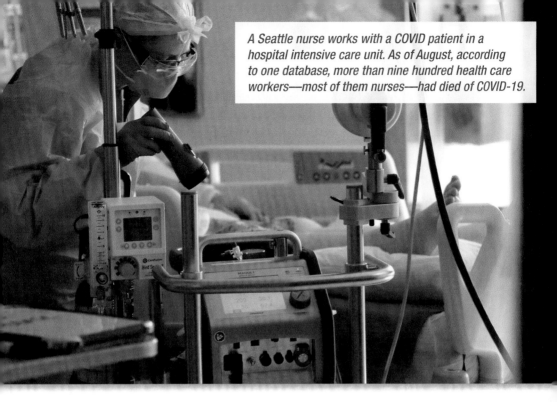

A Seattle nurse works with a COVID patient in a hospital intensive care unit. As of August, according to one database, more than nine hundred health care workers—most of them nurses—had died of COVID-19.

virtual office might be the new normal, she concluded, "It is a future without so many of the small daily pleasantries and weekly catch-ups that make us feel noticed, included and connected—a future that seems pretty lonely."[8]

White-collar workers did not escape job losses either. Though white-collar industries experienced fewer job losses at the beginning, in many instances their unemployment numbers have grown even as other parts of the economy are slowly recovering. Data also suggests that layoffs in white-collar industries will be slower to reverse or are more likely to be permanent. "It will get worse before it gets better—white-collar workers will now bear the brunt,"[9] predicted Yelena Shulyatyeva, an economist.

Back to Work During the Pandemic

The US Department of Labor reported that 4.8 million jobs were added in June 2020. Returning workers faced a new normal. Workplace challenges varied by environment, from factories and offices to retail establishments like restaurants and stores. The CDC released voluntary guidelines to help businesses safely reopen. They included details on everything from evaluating their environment's risks and what to do if an employee got sick to proper use and storage of disinfectants.

Returning workers faced new and evolving safety protocols and practices. In many locations, screening procedures such as routine health questions and temperature checks have become another aspect of the new normal. Masks were required, and hand sanitizer dispensers were prominently located. Many workers underwent safety training, including information about proper hand hygiene, disinfection of shared spaces, social distancing, and interactions with colleagues and customers.

Physical environments were altered at many sites. Restaurants expanded into outdoor space. Some restaurants in cities in Southern California, for example, built exterior dining decks over adjacent parking spaces. In office environments, the much-maligned cubicle was reintroduced as a barrier to the spread of coronavirus. Other workplaces designated shared employee spaces such as meeting rooms, lobbies, and communal kitchens as off limits or restricted the number of occupants.

Work processes, such as on automotive assembly lines, adjusted to keep workers safe. But just days after reopening in late May, Ford Motor Company plants in Chicago, Illinois, and Dearborn, Michigan, closed after workers there tested positive. The shutdown underscored the obstacles manufacturers face as they ramp up reopening.

Finally, some employers have initiated policies to accommodate their older and at-risk workers. Reassigning these workers to jobs with less public contact minimized their risks. Staggering work schedules protected them from potentially crowded conditions.

What's Next?

How workers and workplaces will continue to be affected is unclear. Some new workplace changes may disappear; some may become permanent. But most experts agree that the workplace will never be the same.

CHAPTER TWO

Schools

In the spring of 2020, the coronavirus pandemic forced a near-total shutdown of school buildings in the United States. At their peak, the closures affected at least 55.1 million students in 124,000 US public and private schools. And while it was initially hoped that schools would resume after a brief period, nearly every state soon either ordered or recommended that schools remain closed through the end of the 2019–2020 school year. School closures forced a new normal on everyone connected with schools: students, teachers, administrators, and support staff such as bus drivers, food service workers, and custodians.

Parents also found themselves in circumstances they never imagined. "I literally cried—I was crying all afternoon,"[10] a mother and parent advocate in the Bronx admitted. Overnight, family homes—from spacious suburban spaces to cramped city apartments—became classrooms, cafeterias, gyms, and playgrounds. Parents became teachers, cafeteria workers, counselors, and coaches—even as many worked their day jobs remotely and managed parental responsibilities. Many parents, employed as essential workers, were not available at all.

School Is in Session—Virtually

The nation's 3.7 million public and private school teachers bore the burden of their schools' abrupt closures. In what seemed like an instant, on-site, in-person classroom learning went virtual.

For most school districts, the transition to remote learning was chaotic. Teachers hustled to find effective ways to instruct and interact with students from afar. Many lacked technology training. Quickly mastering digital learning systems, video teaching skills, online student progress assessments, cybersecurity practices, and other components of successful remote learning was a formidable task. Plus, about half of public school teachers have children living at home and were juggling jobs with parenting.

As best they could, teachers tried to re-create their classrooms in real time with online platforms like Zoom and Google Classroom. It was not easy. Small-group learning assignments, like having students pair up to discuss a question, were tricky to implement. John Cherichello, a seventh-grade English teacher, explains how that used to work: "I might pose a big question about the perspective of character in a story and have students draw a connection to their own lives in a pair share."[11] But the transition to Zoom required him to divide his class into separate breakout rooms, or small meetings, making it challenging to observe groups, provide feedback, and keep students on track.

Students also logged in to their new normal with varying degrees of success. Technical difficulties stymied many. Younger students faced navigation, comprehension, and concentration issues, needing significant parental support. Security was another early issue as so-called Zoombombers, or hackers, commandeered classrooms to present pornographic and other offensive images, spew hateful racist language, and cause other malicious disruptions.

The Digital Divide

Some students could not log on at all. The issue, referred to as the digital divide—or who has computers and good internet access and who does not—was thrust into the news. According to the Associated Press, approximately 17 percent of US students do not have access to computers at home, and 18 percent do not have access to broadband internet, creating what is known as "the homework gap."[12]

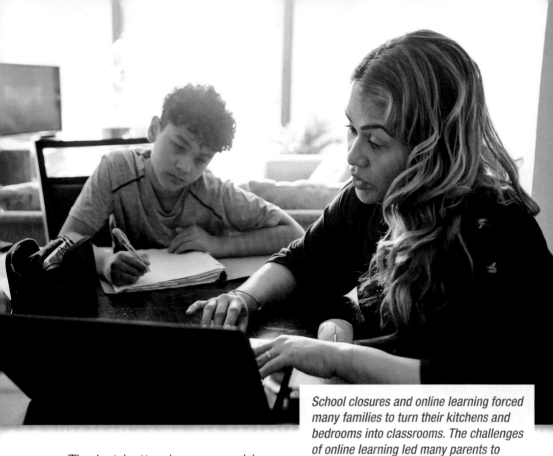

School closures and online learning forced many families to turn their kitchens and bedrooms into classrooms. The challenges of online learning led many parents to take on the role of teacher, even while they did their own jobs from home.

The hot-button issue, a problem long before the COVID-19 crisis, disproportionately impacts Black, Hispanic, Native American, and low-income families, exacerbating existing inequities. In a recent survey of district leaders in high-poverty districts by the Education Week Research Center, more than half cited technology access as a critical challenge to student learning during the shutdown.

Some, mainly bigger, districts bought devices, including laptops and hot spots, and distributed them to students. In Los Angeles, the nation's second-largest school district, one hundred thousand students needed digital devices. Miami-Dade County Public Schools in Florida provided more than eighty thousand mobile devices to students. In numerous cities—including Austin, Texas, and Petal, Mississippi—students connected from their parents' cars to Wi-Fi-wired school buses located in library, church, community center, and apartment house parking lots.

School Outdoors

As COVID-19 spread nationwide, schools grappled with reopening in the fall. Virtual classrooms and in-person learning both raised concerns.

Some schools saw another option for at least partial instruction—moving outdoors. A study from Japan noted that transmission indoors is nearly twenty times more likely than outdoors. And the benefits of being outdoors for students' social, emotional, and mental well-being have long been known.

Some schools stocked up on tents. Others built open-sided shelters. New York City parents called on the mayor to close streets near schools to allow for outside learning.

The idea was not new. In the early part of the twentieth century, open-air schools, an idea pioneered in Germany, launched in the United States to combat tuberculosis, a contagious lung disease. Some classes were even held on roofs or ferries. By 1914 the United States had about 150 open-air institutions in eighty-six cities.

Obstacles to current implementation included funding, leadership opposition, and logistics like transportation and weather. But, advocates warned, "schools need to figure out a new solution because the inside of the building doesn't work as the only solution and online learning doesn't work as the only solution."

Quoted in Erin Einhorn, "Schools Seeking Alternative to Remote Learning Try Experiment: Outdoor Classrooms," NBC News, August 5, 2020. www.nbcnews.com.

Some districts had to rely on low-tech solutions. Isolated rural districts sent home assignment packets through the mail or with school bus drivers wearing protective gear. And only 27 percent of rural districts mandated any actual instruction while schools were closed, according to the Center on Reinventing Public Education, a think tank.

Even as school resumed remotely in the fall, a study by the University of Southern California and the Partnership for Los Angeles Schools revealed the persistence of the digital divide in three Los Angeles minority communities: 17 percent had no internet at home, and 8 percent had mobile internet only. Furthermore, Chase Stafford of the Partnership for Los Angeles Schools noted that the challenges were not unique to the surveyed communities but common to low-income communities nationwide. In Washington, DC, for example, where the 2020–2021 school year also began remotely, many families lacked digital devices (60 percent) and internet access (27 percent) that their children would need for online learning.

Consequences of School Closures

Parents and educators all worried about the effects of the unprecedented academic interruption on students and their communities. Combined with the traditional summer vacation, many schools were closed to in-person learning for at least five months—nearly half of the year. Of greatest concern to both groups was the harm to student learning and achievement.

Education experts point to the well-documented summer learning loss, nicknamed the summer slide, as an example of the potential effects. According to a study by the Northwest Evaluation Association, a nonprofit educational organization, summer learning losses in reading and math are significant. And they get progressively more severe as students get into the higher grades. The organization estimated that students could begin the 2020–2021 school year having lost as much as a third of anticipated progress in reading and half of likely progress in math.

The pandemic's potential learning loss, dubbed the COVID slide, is most likely to affect the most vulnerable students. Ariel Kalil, a professor at the University of Chicago, voiced this dire warning. "Kids who are disproportionately low-income are at highest risk for learning losses. When these gaps in learning open up, absent some really serious and sustained intervention, the kids won't (catch up). That will result in less academic achievement, lower lifetime earnings and even lower productivity in adulthood."[13]

Effects on Social and Emotional Development

For adolescents, school is so much more than six to eight subject periods, pop quizzes, and class projects. There are band rehearsals, sports practice, and spending time with friends in the cafeteria. There are clubs, community service, and student government. US high school students spend on average more than six hours a day in school. With the switch to remote learning, most of them spent that time at home.

Educators and parents speculate that detrimental effects on adolescent growth will not be limited to academics. According to the CDC, long-term school closures are harmful to social and emotional skill development, from learning to make and maintain friendships to how to act in groups. In addition, school provides myriad opportunities for teens to learn to recognize and regulate their emotions, appreciate others' perspectives, interact and form relationships with adults outside their families, set goals, evaluate options, and make good decisions. Acquiring these crucial skills without in-person interactions, experts say, is a tough task.

Plus, missing significant social events, rites of passage like class trips and college visits, senior pranks, prom, and ultimately graduation were real emotional losses for the Class of 2020—3.7 million high school seniors. Joey Graham, a senior athlete, explains, "I've always looked forward to being a senior, and a pretty large chunk of the year is being lost. And it's pretty heartbreaking."[14]

> "I've always looked forward to being a senior, and a pretty large chunk of the year is being lost. And it's pretty heartbreaking."[14]
>
> —Joey Graham, high school senior

Safe at Home?

Sheltering at home, meant to protect children and youth from coronavirus, has potentially put some of them in a dangerous situation. As millions of families struggle with the crisis—illness, iso-

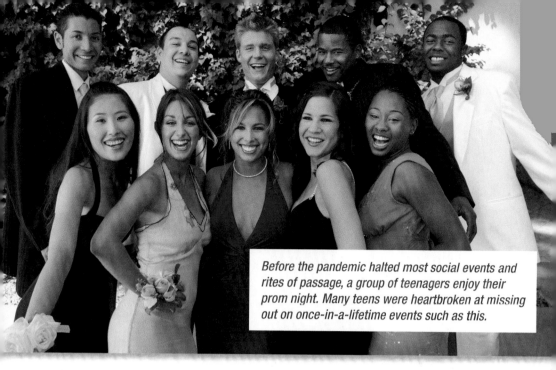

Before the pandemic halted most social events and rites of passage, a group of teenagers enjoy their prom night. Many teens were heartbroken at missing out on once-in-a-lifetime events such as this.

lation, financial problems, stress, and the new demands of having children at home all day—conditions can become overwhelming, and child endangerment may result. Nearly 80 percent of abusers in 2018 were parents, according to a US Department of Health and Human Services report.

Now school closures have cut a lifeline for victims of child abuse and neglect. Nearly 21 percent of child abuse reports are by educators, but since the pandemic began, child abuse reports have plummeted. Shellie McMillon, a children's rights advocate, explains, "One thing we know is that educators, our school professionals, are the largest group of people who report suspected child abuse and that makes sense. They're usually with kids a good portion of the day. Now that kids are not in school, they're at home—a lot of times, they don't have that, what we call a trusted adult, to maybe tell about what's going on."[15]

While maltreatment is the greatest concern, other at-home dangers include risk of accident and injury, excessive screen time, unsafe neighborhoods, exposure to peer pressure, and potential for risky behavior by unsupervised or minimally supervised young people.

Reopening: Rationale and Reservations

These child- and adolescent-welfare worries, as well as economic concerns, prompted calls by various groups, from politicians to pediatricians, to reopen schools. But teachers and parents had mixed feelings about reopening. Public school teachers, one-third of whom are over age fifty, pushed back on in-person reopening. In Tennessee, teachers held mock funeral processions protesting a return to in-person learning. Teachers in San Antonio, Texas, staged a car caravan and symbolic "die-in."

Sixty percent of parents also preferred to delay in-person classes, citing health risks, according to a Kaiser Family Foundation poll published in July. But many other parents were desperate to have their children return to school. Jason Kamras, the schools chief in Richmond, Virginia, described frantic parents who emailed him about losing their jobs and their homes if their kids were not back in school so that they could get back to work.

Still other parents, frustrated and angry that their children were losing yet more months of academic progress and social growth, clamored for schools to reopen. Shalyse Olson, a Salem, Oregon, parent, has been frustrated by the continuation of remote learning into the fall. She started a petition and organized rallies at the state capitol building. Parents held signs proclaiming "School is essential" and "Our kids deserve an education."[16] But in mid-October, the district announced that because county positivity rates were above guidelines, most students would continue to learn remotely until February 2021.

Logistics and Challenges

Despite the ongoing challenges, many schools reopened in the fall, albeit with a patchwork of differing strategies. These included in-person learning, hybrid learning—a mix of in-person and online learning—and full-time remote learning options. According to the Center on Reinventing Public Education, more than half of states and the District of Columbia provided no clear public health guidance for safe school reopening—leaving it to local health authori-

Pandemic Pods

For some mostly affluent families, back-to-school took place in a friend's repurposed living room, a garage, or even a remodeled barn. In so-called pandemic pods, small groups of students in the same grade gathered daily for socialization and learning, usually following virtual lessons from their school districts. In some arrangements, parents supervised the pod on a rotating basis, allowing them work-from-home flexibility. Some pods hired a teacher to manage the pod or to supplement online learning.

But the private pod option was impossible for millions of low-income parents facing the educational, child care, and financial problems posed by the pandemic. Nonprofit organizations such as the YMCA stepped in to provide locations where children could participate in remote learning under staff supervision; meals were often included.

Some school districts also created their own versions of learning pods for eligible groups of students—usually those in need of specific services, such as special education students. So did several municipal governments. In San Francisco the city offered learning hubs for high-needs students— including those who were learning English, homeless, or low income—at libraries and recreation centers. "It will take a village to address the wide range of learning needs for our city's children and youth during the COVID-19 pandemic," said Mayor London Breed.

Quoted in Wyatte Grantham-Phillips, "As School Starts Online, Parents Need to Study Up on 'Pandemic Pods'— and What They Mean for Equity," *USA Today*, July 26, 2020. www.usatoday.com.

ties. Public health experts warned that schools should be prepared for intermittent closures in case of further recurrences.

Most schools that returned to some form of in-person learning faced a new normal. In many, students and staff wore masks. Desks were spaced 6 feet (1.8 m) apart to ensure social distancing. Gathering spaces like cafeterias and courtyards were closed. Recommended symptom screening, intense disinfecting of high-touch surfaces, and limited use of shared equipment and supplies were all disruptive. So were suggestions for staggered school arrival times and alternate seating on school buses. Collaborative learning projects; classes like art, music, and physical education; and extracurricular activities were severely restricted.

While there were difficulties, Mary Coleman was happy to be back in her Long Island classroom. A forty-year veteran teacher, she relies on her district's protocols to protect her. "With masks, social distancing, staggered class dismissal and hand sanitizer in class, I feel very safe," she said. For her, it was a mental health issue. "Frankly, I needed to be back for my own psyche. I need the kids as much as they need me."[17]

Kirill Kilfoyle, a senior at a high school in upstate New York, was also pleased to be back. At his mother's insistence, Kilfoyle began the school year on a hybrid schedule. But when he was allowed to, he grabbed the chance to return to full-time, in-person

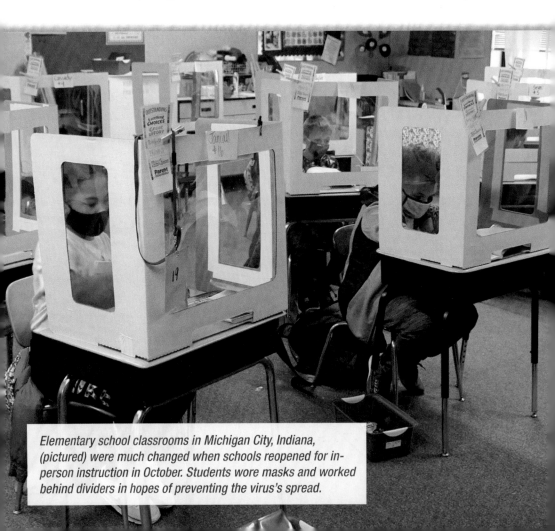

Elementary school classrooms in Michigan City, Indiana, (pictured) were much changed when schools reopened for in-person instruction in October. Students wore masks and worked behind dividers in hopes of preventing the virus's spread.

learning. He said his virtual learning experience in the spring influenced him. "I don't like online learning. When I need it, I can get help in class. When I am home, it is too easy to get distracted. I am trying to have a normal day."[18]

Not everyone was so positive about the return to in-person learning. Carol Flora, a teacher in Lincoln, Nebraska, returned to school to maintain her family's health insurance. She also missed her students, her colleagues, and a "sense of normalcy." But she was not convinced things were back to normal. She worried about getting sick, getting her family sick, and following safety routines, such as cleaning her room between classes. "I worry about everyone and everything. I don't see how . . . students and staff going back to school is logistically going to work."[19] While she returned to her school building, her worries drove her family's decision to choose remote learning for their own three kids, with her husband supervising their boys' virtual schooling at home.

Like the Flora family's children, many students returned to school remotely. According to EdWeek, as of September 22, students in 74 percent of the nation's one hundred largest school districts were returning to school in virtual classrooms. This was occurring even as the hasty spring pivot to remote learning was deemed mostly unsuccessful, with poor attendance being a key issue. In a national survey of 5,659 educators conducted in the spring by Fishbowl, a publication on workplace trends, the majority of teachers said that fewer than half of their students were attending remote classes.

Attendance problems persisted in the fall. Large school districts that started the year virtually—from Dallas and Austin to

> "I don't like online learning. When I need it, I can get help in class. When I am home, it is too easy to get distracted. I am trying to have a normal day."[18]
>
> —Kirill Kilfoyle, high school senior

> "I worry about everyone and everything. I don't see how . . . students and staff going back to school is logistically going to work."[19]
>
> —Carol Flora, teacher

Los Angeles, Nashville, and Philadelphia—all reported enrollment declines. In Detroit only 78 percent of students attended their first week of online class.

Researchers had predicted that hard-to-overcome obstacles would lead to many poor and hard-to-reach students disappearing in the fall. They pointed to factors that included learning disruption, access to materials—especially digital equipment and broadband access—loss of teacher support, and family imperatives such as getting a job and helping with child care. Their prediction was right.

But more affluent families seeking in-person instruction for their children also chose other options, such as joining a learning pod with a private teacher or enrolling in a private school—with those students vanishing from public school rolls. Jennifer Ludtke, a former principal in Las Vegas, Nevada, felt her daughters, ages 12 and 13, had not learned much in the spring. She registered them part time in a local community college program and is staying home to tutor them. Another parent, Melissa Ruiz, could not afford to stay at home with her five-year old son, so she put him in private school, even with the high price tag.

What's Ahead?

The 2020–2021 school year may be just as difficult as the previous one. As the virus surges and subsides, tough choices affecting the future of students, their families, and educators will have to be made.

Significant state and local budget shortfalls and competing priorities threaten to derail schools' recovery. Ensuring adequate investment is critical. Advocates predict federal government funding will be necessary.

And in the classroom, adjustments will continue to be made. Stacy Ward, a Houston-area teacher, no longer has her students chose a high-five, hug, or handshake when they enter her classroom. Instead, they choose between an elbow, a knee, or a foot bump, followed by a squirt of hand sanitizer. "It's normal to them now,"[20] she says.

CHAPTER THREE

Daily Life

On March 13, 2020, President Donald Trump declared a national state of emergency. In the following weeks, the pandemic raced across the nation. Nonessential businesses closed. People hunkered down at home.

Routines, ways of interacting, and pastimes changed. While the changes depended somewhat on where one lived, daily life changed significantly. Leaving home, except for medical appointments, grocery shopping, and exercise, was largely limited. Interacting with others was awkward—no kisses or hugs, no fist bumps or high fives—instead, hand washing was constant. Attending sporting events and concerts, visiting cultural attractions, and enjoying other entertainments gave way to streaming movies at home. From how people dressed to how they dated, the coronavirus upended daily life in ways big and small.

As summer waned and fall arrived, people in various regions of the country tried a return to daily life, even as surges occurred in areas that had previously been mostly spared. According to a report by McKinsey & Company released in October, while 80 percent of Americans felt somewhat unsafe engaging in routine activities, one-third were leaving their homes to participate in so-called normal pursuits.

Businesses in many states have resumed operations, either fully or with some restrictions. As of the beginning of November, an interactive map of businesses maintained and updated regularly by the *New York Times* showed twenty-nine states having reopened, eight states in the process of reopening, six states pausing parts of their reopening, and seven states reversing sectors that had reopened earlier.

Nothing Is Routine Anymore

Accomplishing simple errands and engaging in normal activities has been complicated. Shopping for groceries has required supplies—a mask and hand sanitizer or disinfectant wipes—and a strategic plan—day, time, and place that would minimize waiting in line and contact with others. Many people, especially vulnerable populations, such as senior citizens and individuals with health conditions, have chosen online ordering and home delivery services instead.

Going out for a meal was almost impossible for months as restaurants were shuttered or were open for take-out services only. But by summer, outdoor dining was available in most states. Some states, like Texas, imposed few restrictions on restaurants reopening, including indoor dining. Not all patrons embraced the option to dine indoors. Janice Provost, owner of a Dallas restaurant, noted her patrons' preferences: "Some people are like, absolutely only outside." She strung lights outside like a Parisian café, and she said, "It's a little happy, even if we can't go to Paris right now."[21]

By fall, restaurants in most states, even some with hard-hit cities, were open for indoor dining with varying restrictions, just in time for winter. But Karl Franz Williams, owner of 67 Orange Street in New York City, says the pandemic has made him more comfortable with uncertainty, "The new norm is we don't know what's going to happen when it's going to happen and how it's going to look until it happens."[22]

Personal care establishments, like hair salons, were closed throughout much of the spring and early summer. So shaggy-haired clientele got creative. YouTube became a standby consultant, and individuals, some armed with equipment purchased online, cut and styled their own or family members' hair. As salons reopened, safety measures were prioritized. At some salons, clients have been asked to wait in their cars until their appointment time and undergo a temperature check as they enter. Stylists and clients chat with one another through masks, and many of the added perks—from coffee stations to popular magazines—are gone.

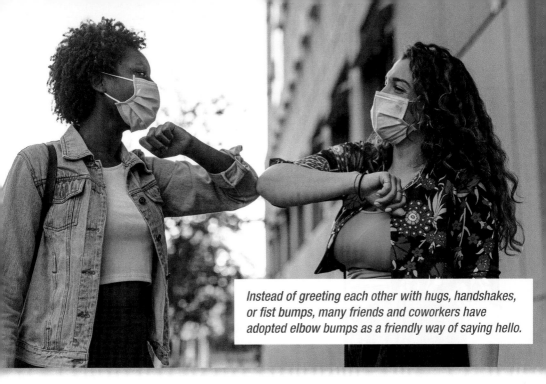

Instead of greeting each other with hugs, handshakes, or fist bumps, many friends and coworkers have adopted elbow bumps as a friendly way of saying hello.

Gyms and fitness centers were barred from opening for months. Among the last businesses to reopen, many gyms have overhauled their operations: closing locker rooms, suspending group classes, instituting temperature checks, spacing out equipment, and sanitizing constantly. Some gyms in Southern California have moved fitness equipment, like stationary bikes, outdoors. But people remain cautious about indoor activities, and many people's fitness habits changed at the pandemic's start. Determined individuals and families took to the outdoors—hiking, biking, and making an outing of walking the dog. Some exercised in virtual fitness classes or stayed a socially safe distance from recently hired personal trainers. Others installed new gym equipment at home.

Living Life Virtually

Much of daily life in 2020 went virtual. Friends and family gathered online via Skype, Google Meet, and Zoom. By summer, Zoom saw explosive growth of more than 300 million daily users, up from 10 million prior to the pandemic. There were Zoom classes, parties, birthday celebrations, book clubs, blind dates, play dates,

Religious Observance

In the midst of the pandemic, limits on public gatherings caused houses of worship to close. Religious observance took new forms. Some congregations met outside on lawns or at the beach or a park. Drive-in religious services popped up in parking lots or by arrangement with drive-in movie theaters.

Cars also facilitated important life cycle events. In Los Angeles one young man celebrated his bar mitzvah—the coming of age service that marks a Jewish boy's thirteenth birthday—with a "carmitzvah" conducted in a rooftop parking lot. Hosts greeted guests from a golf cart. Car selfies were uploaded to a big screen. And when the young man concluded his ritual chanting, honking horns recognized his accomplishment. In Maryland a Muslim community re-created the hajj, a pilgrimage tradition, in a school parking lot. Families followed a brief route with stations symbolizing all the customary rites.

But most religious observance took place virtually. Fifty-seven percent of Americans watched religious services on TV or participated online via websites, social media platforms, and streaming services. Even holiday festivities occurred over Zoom. There were Easter dinners, Ramadan fast-breaking meals, and Jewish seders.

and concerts. According to a Pew Research Center survey in early April, approximately one-third of Americans had attended an online party or gathering. Twenty percent had watched a livestreamed event such as a concert or play. Online fitness classes and workouts had attracted about 18 percent of the population.

Cultural attractions like museums offered online gallery tours and exhibits that patrons could view from the comfort of their couch. Zoos and aquariums focused their cameras on several of their animal areas so visitors could check on their favorites' antics. National parks and botanical gardens welcomed virtual guests as well. As many of these attractions struggle to reopen with limited hours and occupancy restrictions, fewer patrons are visiting, causing funding shortages, layoffs, and appeals to members to make up the slack.

Tara Riemer of the Alaska SeaLife Center in Seward, Alaska, for example, worries that budget shortfalls will mean closing the facility.

As social distancing policies progressively limited gatherings, even rituals recognizing important life cycle events were livestreamed. Funeral services, many being held for virus victims, went virtual, which has devastated grieving families. Weddings, too, were canceled, postponed, or conducted via Zoom or Facebook. While he had no weepy speeches, bulging dessert tables, or attendants, groom Sean Bouvier described his Zoom wedding glowingly: "I wouldn't trade it for the world. It was super intimate. It's a joyous moment in a negative time."[23]

Even many months into the pandemic, it may be too soon to know how many of these changes will be long-lasting, perhaps permanent. Still, after the pandemic is over, according to a Pew Research Center poll in August, slightly more than half (51 percent) of US adults expect their lives to remain changed in major ways. The other half expect a return to normalcy.

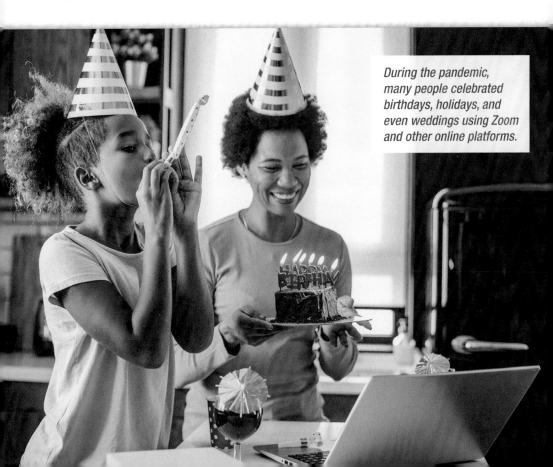

During the pandemic, many people celebrated birthdays, holidays, and even weddings using Zoom and other online platforms.

Stresses on Mental Health

As social distancing forced countless daily routines online, psychologists and social scientists warned of a "social recession,"[24]—the disruption in social connections caused by lengthy periods of isolation. "The irony is that this is happening during a time of extraordinary stress, when our lives are turned upside down," explained Vivek Murthy, former surgeon general of the United States. "Typically, in moments of stress, we reach out to people. We spend time with people we love. And now we're being asked not to do that, at least in physical terms."[25]

Mental health has suffered. In March a Kaiser Family Foundation poll found that 32 percent of US adults reported that their overall mental health had been negatively affected due to virus-related concerns. By mid-July, that number had risen to 53 percent. In addition to anxiety or depression, which rose from 34.5 percent in May to over 40 percent in July, many adults also reported unhealthy changes to routines that affect mental health and well-being: difficulty sleeping, poor eating habits, and increased alcohol or substance abuse. Particularly troubling, nearly 11 percent of respondents in a late June CDC survey reported having seriously considered suicide in the thirty days before the survey.

> "In some ways, this is a perfect storm for mental health issues. We're dealing with social isolation, anxiety around health, and economic problems."[26]
>
> —Jean Twenge, professor

According to professor Jean Twenge, coauthor of a study undertaken by San Diego State University and Florida State University in April, "In some ways, this is a perfect storm for mental health issues. We're dealing with social isolation, anxiety around health, and economic problems."[26]

Vulnerable Populations

The pandemic has dealt a double whammy to older Americans—the danger of contracting COVID-19 and the menace of social isolation to their physical and mental health. Those over age sixty were

Pandemic Pets

Pandemic life can be lonely. The solution for many people during long lockdown days was adopting or fostering a cat or dog. Animal rescue facilities nationwide saw a jump in adoptions and foster care applications at the beginning of the health crisis. "A lot of people are facing prolonged periods of time at home and inside. They want companionship and to not feel alone during this unsettling time," explained Eileen Hanavan, a director at the American Society for the Prevention of Cruelty to Animals.

One adoptive "parent" described his new pet, a dog named Jepsen, this way: "He has brought so much joy into our lives during an otherwise very dark time. Jepsen is a companion for me when I'd otherwise be alone working from home, and taking care of him helps to take my mind off of the seeming constant bad news around us."

Quoted in Sandra E. Garcia, "Foster Pets Are Finding Homes with Quarantined Americans," *New York Times*, March 19, 2020. www.nytimes.com.

Quoted in Amy Wong, "Pandemic Pets: Readers Share Stories About the New Furry Friends They've Adopted," *Seattle Times*, September 2, 2020. www.seattletimes.com.

specifically warned to limit their contacts with others. According to William Schaffner, CDC adviser and infectious disease expert at Vanderbilt University, "The single most important thing you can do to avoid the virus is reduce your face-to-face contact with people."[27]

But humans are social beings. Isolation and loneliness cause stress. According to a National Academies of Sciences, Engineering, and Medicine report, the health consequences of isolation to older adults are profound. They include heightened risk of dementia, stroke, and heart disease among other concerns. As in other populations, mental health risks—depression, anxiety, and suicidal thoughts have also increased.

Although generally healthy and less likely to get seriously ill if they contract the virus, young people have also been impacted by stay-at-home orders and physical distancing constraints. Restricted routines, conflict at home, and worry about world and national affairs, from the pandemic to protests, have compounded the effect. Too much screen time and social media use have further exacerbated the results. Blocked from involvement in their usual whirlwind of social activities—school, clubs, sports, friends, dating—many young people have wound up feeling more isolated, lonely, and depressed.

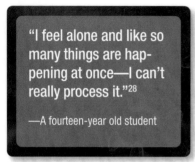

"I feel alone and like so many things are happening at once—I can't really process it."[28]

—A fourteen-year old student

As one fourteen-year-old explained, "I feel alone and like so many things are happening at once—I can't really process it."[28] A September survey of more than two thousand high school and college students reported that almost 75 percent of them said that their mental health had worsened since the beginning of the pandemic, according to Active Minds, a nonprofit organization focused on student mental health. Survey respondents stated that they were experiencing increased stress, loneliness, sadness, and depression.

Disparities

Americans' experience of the pandemic has been shaped by a variety of factors. According to a Pew Research Center study at the end of March, nearly nine in ten US adults said the pandemic has changed their life. Of those who said their life changed, 44 percent said their life changed considerably.

Despite the optimistic signs proclaiming, "We're all in this together,"[29] the pandemic has exposed the nation's extensive economic and race-based inequalities and their enormous effect on how people have weathered the crisis. According to information released by the CDC in August, pandemic-related infections, hospitalizations, and deaths for African Americans, Hispanics, and Native Americans have been significantly higher than for White Americans. Poverty, preexisting health conditions, access to health care, and increased occupational exposure as an essential worker—prevalent in these communities—has heightened the dramatic differences. Samantha Artiga, director of a Kaiser Family Foundation research project on racial disparities, noted, "When you look at that continually growing body of research, the findings very consistently show that people of color are really bearing the heaviest burden of COVID-19 at every stage, from risk of exposure, to access to testing, to severity of the illness and eventually death."[30]

Women have experienced pandemic life differently from men, according to a University of Southern California study. Women have been concerned about a number of issues, including getting food and supplies and the risks of getting sick. Women likewise have reported being lonelier and more anxious. Additionally, women were less positive than men about the quality of their relationships with both their spouse and their children since the pandemic began. Moreover, a variety of factors, from employment in decimated industries to earning lower wages than their husbands, made it more likely that women would lose their jobs or leave the workforce to shoulder child care responsibilities. Emily Janoch, researcher for CARE, an international nonprofit aid organization, found similar results in a study released in September. She explains, "When you ask women if their anxiety has gone up, they say 'Yes, and here's why: I'm not sure how many more days I can feed my family. I'm afraid I'm going to lose my job, and I have no back-up plan."[31]

Reopening Roller Coaster

In May, after nearly two months of pandemic shutdowns, many states partially lifted restrictions. Pressure from the Trump administration and from state and local governments and business groups influenced these decisions. The road to reopening has been a roller-coaster ride.

As Americans resumed some everyday activities, from eating in restaurants to shopping to gathering with friends, COVID-19 cases spiked again. By summer, a surge—driven mostly by states in the South and the West that had led the early drive to ease restrictions—was evident. Florida saw a tenfold case count increase from May. Cases in Texas and Arizona rose 680 percent and 850 percent, respectively, in roughly the same time period.

As a result, many Americans harbored serious doubts about the safety of various activities. Polls by the Democracy Fund and

UCLA Nationscape in June and July showed a drop in the percentage of Americans who felt safe doing routine activities such as going to a concert, movie, sporting event, or restaurant; flying on an airplane; and attending a funeral or wedding.

During the fall, public attitudes toward resuming several popular pastimes, tracked on a weekly basis by Morning Consult, an expert in brands and business trends, rose and fell with the reported cases of the virus. More Americans reported being comfortable with certain pastimes, including dining out (42 percent) and shopping at malls (35 percent). But by the end of October, at least two out of five people said they would not be returning to movie theaters or concert venues, visiting amusement parks, or traveling abroad until at least the spring of 2021.

Infectious disease experts were even less optimistic. A *New York Times* poll of 511 epidemiologists taken in the last week of May asked these professionals when they would resume twenty activities of daily life. Those surveyed said it would take three to twelve months to resume most routine activities, including eating at a dine-in restaurant, sending kids to school, and working in a shared office. It would take a year or more for many to attend religious services, sporting events, weddings, or funerals.

Masks Matter

The epidemiologists surveyed also said it would take more than a year to stop routinely wearing masks. The CDC has recommended that people two years of age and older wear masks in public and around others not living in their household when a distance of 6 feet (1.8 m) cannot be maintained. Masks create a barrier that catches respiratory droplets expelled by an infected individual when the person speaks, sneezes, coughs, or talks and prevents him or her from transmitting the coronavirus to others.

While more than half of states have mask mandates, there is no national mask directive. But in mid-July the CDC called on Americans to wear masks to prevent the virus from spreading. CDC director Dr. Robert R. Redfield stated, "Cloth face coverings are one of the most powerful weapons we have to slow and stop the spread

How Americans Feel About the New Normal

Americans express mixed feelings about life in the new normal, according to a 2020 survey by the Cleveland Clinic and *Parade* magazine. The Healthy Now survey of one thousand adults reveals that many Americans have responded to the pandemic by making healthy lifestyle changes, but many are also experiencing mental health challenges including depression and loneliness. Young adults, in particular, show high percentages in both of these areas. The mixed feelings are perhaps most evident in two other questions: 51 percent of respondents believe that life will never get back to normal, but 72 percent remain hopeful for the future.

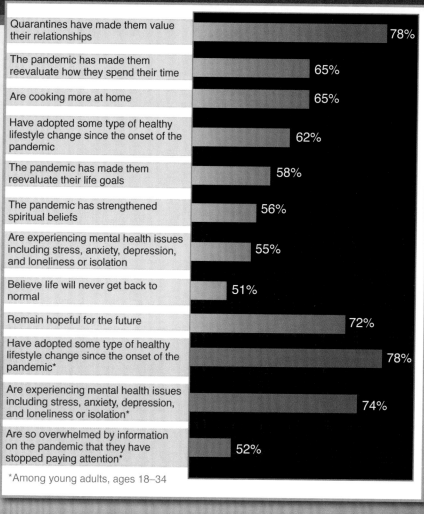

Quarantines have made them value their relationships	78%
The pandemic has made them reevaluate how they spend their time	65%
Are cooking more at home	65%
Have adopted some type of healthy lifestyle change since the onset of the pandemic	62%
The pandemic has made them reevaluate their life goals	58%
The pandemic has strengthened spiritual beliefs	56%
Are experiencing mental health issues including stress, anxiety, depression, and loneliness or isolation	55%
Believe life will never get back to normal	51%
Remain hopeful for the future	72%
Have adopted some type of healthy lifestyle change since the onset of the pandemic*	78%
Are experiencing mental health issues including stress, anxiety, depression, and loneliness or isolation*	74%
Are so overwhelmed by information on the pandemic that they have stopped paying attention*	52%

*Among young adults, ages 18–34

Source: "Parade/Cleveland Clinic Survey Shows Americans Embracing Healthy Lifestyle Changes Amid COVID-19 Pandemic," *Parade* and Cleveland Clinic, September 25, 2020. https://newsroom.clevelandclinic.org/2020/09/25/parade-cleveland-clinic-survey-shows-americans-embracing-healthy-lifestyle-changes-amid-covid-19-pandemic/.

of the virus. . . . All Americans have a responsibility to protect themselves, their families, and their communities."[32]

Masks are a symbol of a divided America. Throughout the pandemic, President Trump has made negative remarks about masks and criticized those who wore them. Many other Republican officials have done the same. Joe Biden, who won the 2020 presidential election, has consistently worn a mask during his public appearances. While wearing one is not a guarantee of political affiliation, research by a team from Syracuse University in July found that political party predicted mask use more than any other factor, with Democrats more likely to wear masks than Republicans.

To many, masks represent their individual sacrifice for the greater good. But others see it as un-American—big government infringing on their personal freedom. "Making individual decisions is the American way,"[33] explains Max Parsell, a power line worker who does not wear a mask.

But sometimes the division spills over into violence. A security guard at a Family Dollar store in Flint, Michigan, was fatally shot by a customer who refused the guard's demand to wear a mask. And two sisters, who allegedly stabbed a store security guard in a shoe store in Chicago twenty-seven times after he told them to put on masks, were arrested on attempted murder charges.

When Will It Be Normal Again?

Daily life in the United States has a long way to go to recover anything resembling normalcy. Surges in infection and uncertainty about the future fuel fears. Asked in October about a return to normalcy, Dr. Anthony Fauci, director of the National Institute of Allergy and Infectious Diseases, said, "I think it will be easily by the end of 2021, and perhaps even into the next year before we start having any semblances of normality."[34]

Still, many Americans remain optimistic. A survey of one thousand adults published in September and conducted by the Cleveland Clinic and *Parade* magazine noted that 65 percent of respondents said they have reevaluated how they spend their time, and 72 percent said they remain hopeful for the future.

CHAPTER FOUR

A New and Different Normal

The coronavirus crisis will eventually end. Experts agree that a combination of factors will likely get the virus under control. A safe, effective vaccine will likely be the most important factor. Continued public health measures—masks and social distancing—will limit transmission until enough people develop immunity to the virus.

But health professionals and researchers are still learning about the virus. They warn that an accurate timeline of its demise is unpredictable. Compliance with public health guidelines regarding masks and social distancing, the availability of rapid COVID-19 tests, the effectiveness of vaccines, and the number of people who choose to be inoculated will all have an effect. Virologist Angela Rasmussen explains, "I don't see this pandemic ending as in like, you know, 'This is the day, the pandemic ended.' I see this as being a process that will go for a long time, potentially even years."[35]

A Vaccine Is Vital

Any end to and recovery from the pandemic will require that a vaccine, or vaccines, be widely available. As of October 2020, more than one hundred coronavirus vaccines were in various stages of development around the world.

Vaccines go through a three-stage clinical trial process before they are sent to regulatory agencies for approval. It can take ten to fifteen years to bring a vaccine to market, but scientists have been sprinting to produce a safe and effective

Pandemics Inspire Progress

Like COVID-19, previous pandemics have brought death and devastation. But they have also led to innovations. According to journalism professor Katherine Foss, "Public policy and society as a whole have been dramatically shaped by epidemics."

In the fourteenth century, the Black Death, or plague, in Europe killed so many of the working poor that their reduced numbers enabled laborers to demand higher wages, better living conditions, and increased freedom. Authorities also realized the effects of poor sanitation, leading to improvements in public systems. The concept of quarantine, from the Italian word *quarantena*, the isolation of ships for forty days, was first implemented as well.

The 1918 flu pandemic took the lives of 50 million to 100 million people worldwide—675,000 in the United States. Mitigation measures still used today—including face masks, hand hygiene, social distancing, and mass closings—were instituted during that pandemic. Significantly, the catastrophe also led to public health policies in the United States and abroad, including ideas about preventive medicine and expanded access to health care through government- or employer-sponsored insurance plans. First-floor bathrooms—which prevented potentially infected delivery persons from using the family's personal bathroom—had their introduction during the crisis.

Quoted in Glenn McDonald, "5 Advances That Followed Pandemics," History, July 15, 2020. www.history.com.

coronavirus vaccine by 2021. In 2020 the US government, through its COVID-19 vaccine research and development program, Operation Warp Speed, committed $10 billion toward the goal of developing and delivering 300 million vaccine doses by January 2021.

While obstacles to achieving that goal were significant, vaccine development has progressed faster than predicted. In November, two highly effective vaccine candidates had been submitted to the Food and Drug Administration (FDA) for emergency use authorization. At least one of them was likely to be approved and available for inoculating small numbers of certain populations—health care professionals, nursing home staff and residents, and some essential workers—in early 2021.

Large-scale and widespread vaccination campaigns still faced substantial hurdles: limited initial supplies, a likely two-dose regimen, and challenging vaccine storage requirements. Misinformation, conspiracy theories, public trust, and antivaccination sentiment in the United States must also be overcome. Harvard professor Yonatan Grad said that even once a vaccine becomes available, "it seems, to me, unlikely that a vaccine is an off-switch or a reset button where we will go back to pre-pandemic times."[36]

Toward a Better Normal

If the experts' predictions are accurate, Americans are going to have to figure out a way to live with coronavirus for the next year and possibly longer. Moreover, leaders and activists from various fields, from science and sociology to education and politics, have pointed to the fact that pre-pandemic times were not working for millions of Americans, including the homeless, the poor, and communities of color.

Many thinkers view the pandemic as an opportunity for big institutional changes, from pandemic preparedness and public health to government and the economy. Science historian Naomi Oreskes notes, "If you look at history, you often see big social change follow from crisis. This is an opportunity for a big change: a reconnection to the idea of a common good, collective responsibility."[37]

"If you look at history, you often see big social change follow from crisis. This is an opportunity for a big change: a reconnection to the idea of a common good, collective responsibility."[37]

—Naomi Oreskes, science historian

Pandemic Preparedness and Public Health

If scientists have waffled on how the pandemic will end, they have been mostly united in their assessment of the country's uneven response to the outbreak and the need for better pandemic

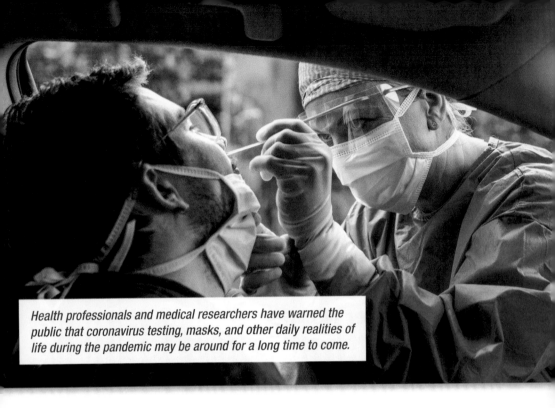

Health professionals and medical researchers have warned the public that coronavirus testing, masks, and other daily realities of life during the pandemic may be around for a long time to come.

preparedness. "The US cannot prepare for these inevitable crises if it returns to normal as many of its people ache to do," writes journalist Ed Yong. "Normal led to this. Normal was a world ever more prone to a pandemic but ever less ready for one. To avert another catastrophe, the US needs to grapple with all the ways normal failed us."[38]

US administrations have struggled with pandemic preparedness for decades. The efforts became more urgent after 9/11 as officials worried about a bioterrorism attack. Uneven progress was made under the Bush and Obama administrations. However, the Obama administration, faced with both the H1N1 and Ebola virus outbreaks, conducted an emergency simulation of an airborne, respiratory virus and developed procedures and a detailed pandemic response playbook.

But the Trump administration simply did not take the threat seriously enough. Documents obtained by the news organization Politico detail a January 13, 2017, session on pandemic preparedness presented by outgoing Obama administration officials to thirty Trump administration senior officials. Furthermore, in 2017 the

Trump team was made aware of the sixty-nine-page "Playbook for Early Response to High-Consequence Emerging Infectious Disease Threats and Biological Incidents," prepared by the National Security Council. Briefed on preparedness status and armed with a pandemic-fighting playbook, the administration largely ignored both. Instead, personnel and funding for agencies and government programs responsible for detecting and responding to a pandemic were slashed. Even in 2019 when the Trump administration's simulation exercise, called Crimson Contagion, revealed that the nation was unprepared for a pandemic, little action was taken. Finally, according to journalist Bob Woodward's book *Rage*, in January 2020 Trump received but dismissed daily intelligence briefings about the impending coronavirus outbreak. Even when he knew how serious the virus was, Trump kept the information from the public. Then he downplayed the disease's impact.

If the pandemic has taught people anything, it is the importance of preparing for the next one. Public health systems—the professionals and agencies that are charged with safeguarding the nation's health—are the front line in researching and responding to infectious disease outbreaks like COVID-19. But the US public health system is severely underfunded. According to the Trust for America's Health, as of 2017, just 2.5 percent of the entire US health care budget was spent on public health. Understaffing in critical public health positions likewise threatens the delivery of emergency services. A Kaiser Health News and Associated Press analysis found that local health departments have thirty-eight thousand fewer employees since the 2008 recession. Bolstering public health agency funding and personnel will be required to ensure a better outcome when the next pandemic strikes.

Experts also warn that pandemic preparedness measures are inadequate. Infrastructure improvements to respond to the next pandemic include identifying, stockpiling, and managing essential medical supplies, such as ventilators and protective equipment, on the national level. Capacity for rapid, efficient development and manufacture of accurate, widely available diagnostic tests, antiviral medications, and ultimately vaccines must also be addressed. In addition, a federal government plan to coordinate the distribution of supplies and equipment in a fair, well-organized, effective manner must also be created.

Universal Health Care: A Fundamental Right

The coronavirus crisis exposed a US public health system that was inadequate to respond to a pandemic. But it also revealed issues of inadequate health insurance coverage and unequal access to health care services. Representative Pramila Jayapal of Washington State is among those who say that there is a need for significant health care reform. She states, "I hate to say we needed a crisis like this because it has caused so much devastation, but certainly the crisis has highlighted the human toll of our broken health-care system."[39]

In the United States most individual health care services—such as doctors' visits, medical procedures, hospitalization, and medications—are paid for partially or in full by private insurance companies. About half of Americans get this valuable benefit through their employers. This leaves the other half, including underemployed, unemployed, and part-time workers, without access to medical care or with crushing medical bills.

Americans face higher out-of-pocket costs for their medical care than citizens of almost any other country, and even insured individuals often encounter whopping medical care costs. Financial hardship causes many people to delay care or to dispense with treatment altogether. Such actions have dangerous consequences for individuals in ordinary times. During a pandemic, the impact on communities can be devastating. Wendell Potter, a former executive of a health insurance company, explains, "People without insurance (28 million of us) often skip needed care. With coronavirus, this means potentially infected people won't seek testing, let alone treatment—which also means an infected person who goes untreated could help spread the disease to many others."[40]

Pandemics and Protests

On May 25, 2020, George Floyd, an African American man, was killed by four Minneapolis police officers. Floyd had been detained on suspicion of a misdemeanor, but the situation escalated. One officer restrained a handcuffed Floyd with a knee on his neck despite Floyd's pleas that he could not breathe.

Floyd's subsequent death, caught on police bodycam, but also caught on cell phone video by onlookers and spread through social media, prompted massive, often violent, street protests across the United States even amid pandemic fears. "The police violence against black people—that's a pandemic too," said a community organizer in Miami. Further fueling the protests was anger over long-standing economic, social, and health care disparities, exposed by the community's disproportionate coronavirus deaths and job losses.

One group of protesters was health professionals. They had a clear message: racism is a public health crisis. Twelve hundred of them signed a letter supporting the protests. It also called for efforts to alleviate the risks of spreading the virus at gatherings where thousands of passionate protesters are yelling, chanting, and cheering. It stated in part, "We support (racial-justice protests) as vital to the national public health and to the threatened health specifically of Black people in the United States."

Quoted in Julie Bosman and Amy Harmon, "Protests Draw Shoulder-to-Shoulder Crowds After Months of Virus Isolation," *New York Times*, June 2, 2020. www.nytimes.com.

Quoted in Jamie Ducharme, "'Protest Is a Profound Public Health Intervention.' Why So Many Doctors Are Supporting Protests in the Middle of the COVID-19 Pandemic," *Time*, June 10, 2020. https://time.com.

Many health care professionals, policy makers, and activists believe the solution to this challenge is the provision of comprehensive health care as a universal right. According to a 2018 Pew Research Center survey, six in ten Americans believe it is the federal government's responsibility to make sure all Americans have health care coverage. Universal health care, a system in which the government guarantees coverage for everyone and oversees costs, is seen in most of the developed world.

But in the United States, universal health care coverage is a hotly debated proposition. Republicans largely point to the astronomical costs of providing health care for millions. Democrats largely point to universal health care's social equity and economic security benefits. Partisanship and significant division over the issue make resolution unclear. However, the pandemic has put health care center stage, and many health reform advocates remain optimistic.

Economic Inequality

The public health crisis has resulted in a correspondingly devastating economic crisis. At least 45 million people have filed for unemployment since the pandemic began. A US Census Bureau survey in September 2020 found that nearly 23 million adults live in households in which there was not enough to eat in the previous seven days.

In contrast, US household wealth grew nearly 7 percent between April and June, according to a September Federal Reserve report. The gains, secured by the most affluent Americans, underline the nation's expanding economic inequality. In 2019, even before the pandemic, the US Census Bureau found that income inequality, the gap between rich and poor, was at its highest level in fifty years. "The pandemic has only laid bare inequities that have existed in our country for a long time,"[41] said Tara Raghuveer, a housing rights activist.

The pandemic put essential, frontline workers—from health care providers and farmworkers to grocery and postal clerks to bus and delivery drivers—in the spotlight. Declared heroes, in some cities they were applauded nightly. But this celebration stands in stark opposition to their distressed economic lives. Most essential workers live at the bottom of the income ladder. Nationally, essential workers earn an average of 18.2 percent less than employees in other industries, according to Business.org, a consulting group. Research by the Brookings Institution found that wages for home health and personal care workers are so low that nearly 20 percent of care workers live in poverty and more than 40 percent are on some form of public assistance. According to

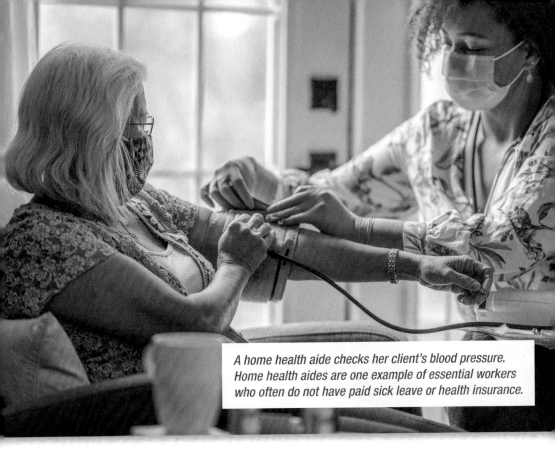

A home health aide checks her client's blood pressure. Home health aides are one example of essential workers who often do not have paid sick leave or health insurance.

economist Gene Sperling, almost half of nursing and home health care aides do not get paid sick leave either. Finally, one in seven essential workers lacks health care insurance altogether; many others are underinsured, facing potentially crushing expenses.

Establishing a fair minimum wage, paid sick leave, and universal health care security, actions that could dramatically improve economic inequality, all require policy decisions that have mixed support among lawmakers, employers, and the general public. However, the pandemic's immense pain and suffering might force a reckoning over the deep divisions and immense societal inequities in the United States.

The Role of Government

Some policy makers question whether the pandemic's toll will have lasting effects on national politics. The pandemic has prompted intense public discussion, even mass protests, of flaws in US systems: extreme economic inequality, huge health care disparities, the digital divide. While many government pandemic relief efforts—writing checks to suffering workers, expanding unemployment benefits and paid sick leave, and delivering billions in business bailouts—were temporary emergency measures, they have been popular with the public.

This widespread approval of significant government intervention may signal a shift in the role Americans want government to assume. David Paleologos of the Suffolk University Political Research Center explains the results of a poll he conducted in April: "The poll shows that when people need help, they can quickly change their ideas about 'big government' . . . with the pandemic threatening lives and livelihoods, we are seeing more people willing to listen to government officials and take advantage of assistance than we've seen in our lifetimes."[42] The debate over the size and scope of government has been at the center of American politics for decades. It is one of the defining differences between Democrats and Republicans. The crisis has energized Democrats who believe the federal government has fundamental essential obligations to its citizens. Democratic senator Chris Van Hollen observes, "What this emergency has done is . . . expose the deep divides in the country, many of the inequities in the country and many of the shortcomings in our systems. The next question will be whether we will muster the political will to use government to address some of these fundamental challenges."[43]

> "What this emergency has done is . . . expose the deep divides in the country, many of the inequities in the country and many of the shortcomings in our systems."[43]
>
> —Chris Van Hollen, US senator

Republican advocates of limited government, however, are determined that a return to pre-pandemic conditions occurs. "I certainly hope that [the pandemic] does not reshape or dramatically expand the role of government in the long term," said Republican senator Patrick J. Toomey. "I think this is a necessary step for an absolutely unique set of circumstances. But I think this is a very, very rare moment. . . . I'm hoping that we return as close as possible to normal."[44]

But a *Wall Street Journal*/NBC News poll conducted in the spring of 2020 found that two-thirds of those surveyed, regardless of political party, approved of the government's expanded role during the COVID-19 crisis. It remains to be seen, however, whether the coronavirus crisis results in political changes that reduce social and economic inequities.

What's Next?

The United States will be living with COVID-19 and its consequences for years to come. It is possible that what has been learned will enable a more just, more equal, and better normal to emerge from the crisis. Former surgeon general Vivek Murthy suggests:

> If we use this moment to recognize that to build lives centered around people, and to make the case for creating a people-centered society—where we think about human connection as we design workplaces and schools, where we think about human connection when we're assessing the impact of policy as well—then I think we will put ourselves on the path to creating a society that is healthier and stronger, but also more resilient, than before the pandemic began.[45]

Introduction: The Crisis Begins

1. Quoted in Maegan Vazquez and Caroline Kelly, "Trump Says Coronavirus Will 'Disappear' Eventually," CNN, February 27, 2020. www.cnn.com.

Chapter One: The Workplace

2. Quoted in Yadira Lopez, "The Hospitality Business May Not Come Back for Years. What Will Its Workers Do?," *Miami (FL) Herald*, October 9, 2020. www.miamiherald.com.
3. Quoted in Alisha Haridasani Gupta, "Why Some Women Call This Recession a 'Shecession,'" *New York Times*, May 9, 2020. www.nytimes.com.
4. Quoted in Andrea Hsu, "'This Is Too Much': Working Moms Are Reaching the Breaking Point During the Pandemic," NPR, September 29, 2020. www.npr.org.
5. Dhruv Khullar, "The Essential Workers Filling New York's Coronavirus Wards," *New Yorker*, May 1, 2020. www.newyorker.com.
6. Quoted in Catherine Thorbecke, "'Heroes or Hostages?': Communities of Color Bear the Burden of Essential Work in Coronavirus Crisis," ABC News, May 22, 2020. https://abcnews.go.com.
7. Quoted in *Time*, "'I've Never Been So Afraid.' Employees on the Everyday Terror of Working in Grocery Stores During the Pandemic," April 9, 2020. https://time.com.
8. Ashley Fetters, "Your Work Friends Knew Exactly What Kind of Week You'd Had," *New York Times*, October 21, 2020. www.nytimes.com.
9. Quoted in Joseph Zeballos-Roig, "Up to 6 Million White-Collar Workers Could Lose Their Jobs in Another Wave of Cuts as Coronavirus Fallout Spreads," Business Insider, June 3, 2020. www.businessinsider.com.

Chapter Two: Schools

10. Quoted in Victoria Bekiempis, "'I Literally Cried': Parents Grapple with Impact of US School Closures," *The Guardian* (Manchester, UK), March 16, 2020. www.theguardian.com.

11. Quoted in Suzanne Labarre, "Zoom Is Failing Teachers. Here's How They Would Redesign It," *Fast Company*, September 3, 2020. www.fastcompany.com.

12. Associated Press, "Analysis Indicates Millions of Students Lack Home Internet to Do Homework," Education Week, June 18, 2019. www.edweek.org.

13. Quoted in Grace Hauck, "Some Parents Want to Hire Tutors, Start Mini Schools This Year. Most Can't Afford To," *USA Today*, August 2, 2020. www.usatoday.com.

14. Quoted in Joe Heim, "For High School Seniors, Coronavirus Brings a Sad Ending and Unexpected Lessons," *Washington Post*, March 31, 2020. www.washingtonpost.com.

15. Quoted in Lili Zheng, "Fort Worth Hospital Sees Spike in Severe Child Abuse Cases Over Last Week," NBC DFW, March 21, 2020. www.nbcdfw.com.

16. Quoted in Katie Reilly, "Some Parents Are Demanding In-Person Schooling as the Pandemic Stretches On," *Time*, October 23, 2020. www.time.com.

17. Quoted in Valerie Strauss, "Going Back to School: The Good, the Bad, and the Ugly," *Washington Post*, October 6, 2020. www.washingtonpost.com.

18. Quoted in Strauss, "Going Back to School."

19. Quoted in Margaret Reist, "Going Back to School: One Teacher's Decision in a Pandemic," *Lincoln (NE) Journal Star*, August 31, 2020. https://journalstar.com.

20. Quoted in Aliyya Swaby and Emma Platoff, "Many Texas Students Will Return to Classrooms on Tuesday. Little Will Be Normal," Texas Tribune, September 8, 2020. www.texastribune.com.

Chapter Three: Daily Life

21. Quoted in Taylor Adams, "Dining Out During a Pandemic: 'Absolutely Only Outside,'" *Dallas (TX) Observer*, August 11, 2020. www.dallasobserver.com.

22. Quoted in Camille Petersen, "Indoor Dining Returns to NYC but Restaurants Face Uncertain Fall and Winter," NPR, September 10, 2020. www.npr.org.

23. Quoted in Lavanya Ramanathan, "Virtual Weddings Were No Gimmick for These Couples," Vox, June 24, 2020. www.vox.com.

24. Ezra Klein, "Coronavirus Will Also Cause a Loneliness Epidemic," Vox, March 12, 2020. www.vox.com.

25. Quoted in Vivek Murthy and Pooja Kumar, "Avoiding a 'Social Recession': A Conversation with Vivek Murthy," McKinsey & Company, June 9, 2020. www.mckinsey.com.
26. Quoted in Markham Heid, "COVID-19's Psychological Toll: Mental Distress Among Americans Has Tripled During the Pandemic Compared to 2018," *Time*, May 7, 2020. www.time.com.
27. Quoted in Klein, "Coronavirus Will Also Cause a Loneliness Epidemic."
28. Quoted in Dan Levin, "In a World 'So Upside Down,' the Virus Is Taking a Toll on Young People's Mental Health," *New York Times*, May 20, 2020. www.nytimes.com.
29. Quoted in Antonio Guterres, "We Are All in This Together: Human Rights and COVID-19 Response and Recovery," United Nations, April 23, 2020. www.un.org.
30. Quoted in Daniel Wood, "As Pandemic Deaths Add Up, Racial Disparities Persist—and in Some Cases Worsen," NPR, September 23, 2020. www.npr.org.
31. Quoted in Jeffrey Kluger, "The Coronavirus Pandemic's Outsized Effect on Women's Mental Health Around the World," *Time*, September 24, 2020. www.time.com.
32. Quoted in Centers for Disease Control and Prevention, "CDC Calls on Americans to Wear Masks to Prevent COVID-19 Spread," July 14, 2020. www.cdc.gov.
33. Quoted in Lori Rozsa et al., "The Battle Over Masks in a Pandemic: An All-American Story," *Washington Post*, June 19, 2020. www.washingtonpost.com.
34. Quoted in Madeline Holcombe et al., "US May Not Be Back to Normal Until 2022, Fauci Says," CNN, October 28, 2020. www.cnn.com.

Chapter Four: A New and Different Normal

35. Quoted in Elizabeth Ralph, "Here's How the Pandemic Finally Ends," Politico, September 25, 2020. www.politico.com.
36. Quoted in Carolyn Y. Johnson, "A Coronavirus Vaccine Won't Change the World Right Away," *Washington Post*, August 2, 2020. www.washingtonpost.com.
37. Quoted in Politico, "Coronavirus Will Change the World Permanently. Here's How," March 19, 2020. www.politico.com.
38. Quoted in Ed Yong, "How the Pandemic Defeated America," *The Atlantic*, August 4, 2020. www.theatlantic.com.

39. Quoted in Paige Winfield Cunningham, "The Health 202: Coronavirus Proves U.S. Needs Medicare for All, Its Advocates Say," *Washington Post*, May 26, 2020. www.washingtonpost.com.
40. Quoted in Megan Henney, "Does Coronavirus Outbreak Make a Case for Medicare-for-All?," Fox Business, March 9, 2020. www.foxbusiness.com.
41. Quoted in CBS News, "Income Inequality, and Coronavirus' Economic Fallout," September 6, 2020. www.cbsnews.com.
42. Quoted in Susan Page, "USA TODAY/Suffolk Poll: Support for Big Government Rises to Record Levels amid Coronavirus Crisis," *USA Today*, April 28, 2020. www.usatoday.com.
43. Quoted in Dan Balz, "Government Is Everywhere Now. Where Does It Go Next?," *Washington Post*, April 19, 2020. www.washingtonpost.com.
44. Quoted in Balz, "Government Is Everywhere Now."
45. Murthy and Kumar, "Avoiding a 'Social Recession.'"

Centers for Disease Control and Prevention (CDC)

www.cdc.gov/coronavirus/2019-ncov

The CDC is the nation's premier public health protection agency. The agency's website devotes significant space to coronavirus and COVID-19 facts and statistics. The site also has extensive information on who is at risk, protective measures, contact tracing, community response, schools and youth, and more.

Johns Hopkins Coronavirus Resource Center (CRC)

https://coronavirus.jhu.edu

The CRC, created and run by Johns Hopkins University & Medicine, is a continuously updated source of COVID-19 data and expert guidance. The center gathers and analyzes statistics and other information related to COVID-19 cases, testing, contact tracing, and vaccine research. The site also provides links to numerous articles from a variety of sources.

National Institute of Allergy and Infectious Diseases (NIAID)

www.niaid.nih.gov

The NIAID is one of the twenty-seven institutes and centers that make up the National Institutes of Health. Its website includes information about coronaviruses, the public health and government response to COVID-19, and treatment guidelines. It also provides details on volunteering for prevention clinical studies.

National Institutes of Health (NIH)

www.nih.gov/coronavirus

Part of the US Department of Health and Human Services, the NIH is the largest biomedical research agency in the world. Its website provides information on development of COVID-19 vaccines, testing, and treatments as well as links to other related topics.

US Food & Drug Administration (FDA)

www.fda.gov

The FDA regulates drugs, medical devices, and other products and oversees food safety. Its website provides pandemic-related statistics and information on protective equipment, treatments, and testing. It includes an extensive section of frequently asked questions about a variety of COVID-19 topics.

World Health Organization (WHO)

www.who.int/emergencies/diseases/novel-coronavirus-2019

Working within the framework of the United Nations, the WHO directs and coordinates global health issues. Its website features rolling coronavirus updates, situation reports, travel advice, facts about preventive measures such as masks, information on how the virus spreads, and more.

Additional resources: City, county, and state public health departments

Books

Nicholas A. Christakis, *Apollo's Arrow: The Profound and Enduring Impact of Coronavirus on the Way We Live*. New York: Hachette, 2020.

Bill Hayes, *How We Live Now: Scenes from the Pandemic*. New York: Bloomsbury, 2020.

Hal Marcovitz, *The COVID-19 Pandemic: The World Turned Upside Down*. San Diego, CA: ReferencePoint, 2021.

Klaus Schwab and Thierry Malleret, *COVID-19: The Great Reset*. Zurich, Switzerland: Agentur Schweiz, 2020.

Internet Sources

Angus Chen, "How to Navigate the 'New Normal' of the Pandemic, According to Experts," WBUR, October 5, 2020. www.wbur.org.

Matt Craven et al., "Not the Last Pandemic: Investing Now to Reimagine Public-Health Systems," McKinsey & Company, July 13, 2020. www.mckinsey.com.

Richard Florida, "The Lasting Normal for the Post-Pandemic City," Bloomberg CityLab, June 24, 2020. www.bloomberg.com.

Politico, "Coronavirus Will Change the World. Here's How," March 19, 2020. www.politico.com.

Washington Post staff, "Asked and Answered: What Readers Want to Know About Coronavirus," *Washington Post*, November 6, 2020. www.washingtonpost.com.

Ed Yong, "How the Pandemic Defeated America," *The Atlantic*, August 4, 2020. www.theatlantic.com.

INDEX